CANCER IS NOT THE END

Things I Wish Someone Had Told Me, Breast Cancer Survival and Thriving

By

Claudia J Sarbieski

Copywrite July 10, 2022, by Claudia J Sarbieski

This book is dedicated to:

To my beloved husband, Peter whose love for me was so strong, he loved me through it. To my four children, who are and have always been the lights of my life. It is because of them, and their futures I dug in. To my parents, who gave me love and a life.

And my God, whom without I would not be here.

Table of Contents

Introduction 1

PART I: Is This a Joke? 2

      Chapter One: The Beginning 3

      Chapter Two: Let The Walk Begin 10

      Chapter Five: The Future 19

Epilogue/Conclusion 24

Bibliography 25

Acknowledgments 26

About the Author 27

Introduction

Thank you for taking the time to read this book.

The topic of breast cancer (any cancer really) is something that makes most people uncomfortable. My hope is that this book will help you or a loved one realize that you are not alone!

Cancer is not the end. For many, it is a beginning. We all need to find our purpose and make that the focus during our recovery.

I am a proud four-year survivor and thriver (and counting!) Did I always feel positive? No, I did not. We all have good days and bad days. Where you are is okay. But try and find the silver lining every day. I have found that my recovery was better when I stayed as positive as I could. A wise person once told me, "God only gives you enough grace for the day you are in, no more, no less." I have remembered that and shared it often with others.

Do I have all the answers? No, I do not, only God does. What I do have is my experience and I hope you will take something from my story and use it in a positive way.

Please read and share with anyone who is living the warrior life.

PART I: Is This a Joke?

Chapter One: The Beginning

Most women can relate to what I am going to say next. Men, you may be uncomfortable… but you should know this. Every year, we go for a mammogram. Every year we act like it is the worst thing that can happen to us. Women we know there are way more invasive procedures that we have done than this, dare I say pap smear? But I digress. Every year we get our gumption up, make the appointment and get our cookies, tatas, bazingas… checked.

Our breasts get smashed by the machine, handled by a stranger while we look up at the ceiling and pretend that it's no big deal. However, this procedure, the mammogram can and does save countless lives every year.

In July of 2018, I was late getting mine. I had been like clockwork prior to this. Multiple times I had been told that I had "dense breast" (for those that have not heard this term before, it means that the breast tissue has a rather high amount of glandular tissue, as well as fibrous connective tissue, very little fat). But this, the year I turned 50, I procrastinated. As it turns out, that may have saved my life. please don't postpone your mammogram because of what happened with me, my story is just that… my story.

I entered the facility in July, checked in as usual, and went to the nice pink section reserved especially for mammogram and ultrasound patients. I changed into the short robe that every girl craves to put on. And patiently waited for my name to be called. The tech called my name. We entered the usual room, but a new machine was present, this is why I say my procrastination saved my life. This new machine was capable of detecting irregularities far better than the old technology. Newly installed, this 3-D mammogram machine was impressive had I gone in for my regular visit, there is a chance my cancer would have been missed and by the time my next mammogram rolled around, it would have been a dire situation. The tech and I chatted while she took the images (she remembered me). However, in the middle of the conversation she got a look on her face and said, "we need to take a few more photos." We did that, she then ushered me back to the waiting room. And I waited, and waited, and waited. Ladies came and went from the pink room, ladies that had come in after me, one of them looked at me with pity and issued a "good luck to you" before she exited. This stranger had felt it was necessary to wish me luck, it was at this point; I knew there was trouble.

The tech called me into another room and said, "we have found something suspicious; we need you to have a biopsy asap. Let us schedule that now." I said, "can I go home and get my appointment book?" She looked at me and said, "Lets schedule it now, Dr Mary gets back Wednesday, she's the best we will put you on her schedule." So many thoughts going through my head.

1.   Shit

2.   This is a mistake; they have someone else's image. It will be fine.

3.   What am I going to tell Pete and the kids?

4.   Oh Lord, what am I going to tell my dad!? I know, I am not telling my dad, Pete's telling my dad. He is also telling Audrey. He might be telling everyone.

5.   I have so many things I want to do, this cannot be happening!! WTH

So that fast. An appointment was made with Dr Mary, and off to the races we started. Now in my head I was waffling. Do I tell anyone? What if it turns out to be nothing, and here, I worried the whole gang over nothing? It was tricky. My first mistakes started here. I chose to be light and fluffy. No big deal. All is well. So, I told my husband, my older son, twenty-nine and older daughter, twenty-six. I also said I could go to the biopsy by myself (no big deal). We would keep the younger boys out of it until we had something for sure to worry them with. Gehrig was to be a high school senior in the fall and Jackson was a junior.

I sent everyone off to work/school, and off I went to get my biopsy with Dr. Mary. The care this woman took in explaining everything, showing me everything, numbing everything… made the whole experience the best it could be. My advice? If you do not have a good vibe from ANY of the doctors, get a new one!!!   Dr. Mary informed me about the seeds being placed, they would be used later if the spots ended up being cancerous. I have said this multiple times, it was fascinating. I wish I had not had to experience it, but watching the technology was something… and I realized just how far we had come, years ago women would not have had this. I found myself feeling grateful for not the last time during the experience. When she had finished getting the six samples, she told me she would get back to me as soon as the results came in. I thanked her and went to work.

The next day was rough. Going to work and doing things at home, while the players you are interacting with do not know what you're going through, it was all so emotional. We had our niece's graduation party, surrounded by loved ones, none of whom knew what was going on. I found myself holed up helping in the kitchen, it helped, kept me busy, and I did not have to have long conversations with anyone that could potentially end up with me in unexplained tears. Looking around the room, I wondered, would I be able, or even here, to celebrate the graduations of my two boys? If I could go back… I would have informed my employer, who also happens to be my brother-in-law and is amazingly supportive, as well as my inner circle. My entire family could have used the support and prayers of those we loved sooner than we got them.

The following day was the day we were supposed to get the results, my husband went to the office and my daughter worked from home to get the results with me. The results came. And I had cancer.

The choices I made at this time are ones that I would like a "do over" on. I decided to tell Pete and Patrick over the phone. When Gehrig and Jackson came home from school… I just told them at the kitchen counter. I did not give them a chance to really voice anything. I just said, "everything is going to be fine" and that was that. If I could go back, I would have had a family meeting. I would have let us all lean into each other and voice whatever feelings anyone had, given anyone the floor to say whatever they needed to. I robbed all of them of that. I suggest you do not. I think it would have made for a healthier process for all of us.

When Dr. Mary had called with the results, she also had the names of all the doctors I would need to be in contact with or who would be contacting me asap.

1. Oncologist

2. General surgeon

3. Plastic surgeon

All of this moves at the speed of light. When I was diagnosed, it was the third week of July. I was in to see the oncologist, Dr K within a few days, and the surgeons Dr R and Dr B shortly after. One of my favorite stories and it is something I will never forget. Was my first visit to the oncologist, my intake visit. We sat in the waiting room, Pete, Emily, and I. I looked around the room, people in various stages of treatment. My eyes landed on a woman who was wearing a turban, obviously to hide the fact that she had lost her hair. I again know this is going to sound crazy, but the thought of losing my hair, scared me more than losing a body part. Why do you ask? I think back now, and I know it is because when something so obvious as hair missing is in front of people, they could change how they acted toward me. And that is something I could not manage, pity. The nurse called my name, took me back, and started getting my information. She stopped, turned, gave me a hug, looked me dead in the eyes and said, "we got you." It was then, I cannot explain it, but I knew that God had me, and I was going to be okay no matter what. Dr K asked me what I wanted to do as far as a plan. I said, "you do what you need to. I have the weddings of my children to plan and attend, graduation parties to throw, and grandbabies yet to be born to love." Also, the biggest thing in the back of my head, and it makes me want to cry every time I think about it... I want to grow old with Pete. I want to dance at our children's weddings and hold hands on the beach and watch the sun set, all the sunsets. It sounds corny. I want to have more TIME, which is what must run through the mind of each person diagnosed with a disease that is life threatening, this could steal time. Funny how situations like these make you quickly evaluate what is important, what is not, and what you will do if you are given a chance to have more time.

We had a brief meeting with the general surgeon Dr B. And a much more detailed meeting with Dr R, who was the plastic surgeon. The plan put in place was that the general surgeon would work first, remove all the breast tissue from the breast as well as a sentinel lymph node, I was having immediate reconstruction, so after Dr B. finished his portion, Dr R would come in and do his portion of the job, the reconstruction, considered a complex procedure, the implants placed skin stretched because some needed to be removed, and the incision closed. Tubes are then sewn into place and attached to drainage bulbs.

The first meeting with Dr. R was with Pete, Emily, and I. The second meeting was just me. I did not think I needed to have anyone with me for it, I thought we would just be going over the same things we had at the first appointment. However, it took a turn. My gratitude for Nurse Jamie, on this, and on more than one occasion, she was ready with a smile and whatever I needed. At this appointment you see, I had to choose the implant. She placed various types in my hand. I do not know what it was about holding these "things" that set me off, but the waterworks started. And there I was, alone and crying. Nurse Jamie brought me tissues and let me have a few minutes to collect myself.

I signed the paperwork, and all that was left was the wait, the surgery was the next.

I felt good about the team of doctors we had assembled, but to make my family happy, I went for a second opinion at a well-known hospital in Chicago, a hospital that my family was familiar with. It is because of this experience; I tell you to walk away if you do not get the warm fuzzies from your doctor.

When My husband, daughter and I got to the hospital, I had to redo the mammogram.... Something I truly did not understand. But I went along with the program. Now, I had to run around the week prior to get all the test results including the mammogram to send down to the hospital. I was told the doctor would review everything prior to our appointment, so I express mailed all the information, including the biopsy. It was clear that she had not reviewed a thing when we sat down in the exam room… When my husband asked questions… (which I highly recommend you come with a list of all questions you have! You have a right to understand your treatment AND what is going on with your condition, it is their job to facilitate this) she made a point to look like she was put out by his efforts to understand what was going on with his wife. Now let me just state, my husband is, in my eyes, one of the most intelligent humans I know. That this person, Dr, or no made him feel like he was not asking pertinent questions was a major turnoff to all parties concerned. While he was asking questions, and she was doing this, Emily and I side eyed each other, both giving a face the other knew the meaning of, "is she really acting the way we think she is." When I told her that she was not saying anything different to us than what my team already had, and that I had a surgery date scheduled, she again seemed irritated and became dismissive. She wanted our business, and she was not getting it, she could not understand why we were not choosing her.

My gut told me I had the right doctors already and that was that.

So, there was this gap, about two weeks before surgery. I needed to get things in order. I found myself trying to sort things and throw things away, just wanting things to be in order for the family "just in case.

My eldest, Patrick, had just met a girl (I knew this one was someone special because he kept pretty quiet unless he really liked them), he had a twinkle in his eye, and he wanted us to meet her. I was thrilled and again found myself looking up at the heavens thanking God.

We spent family time together, went to a Journey/Def Leppard concert that was to this day, one of the best days of my life. We met Patrick's girl, Amanda, and she slid into the family dynamic, and we now cannot imagine our lives without her. But for me, I still felt like I had something unfinished, something I needed to do. I had written letters to my loved ones. I had shown Pete who got what if something happened to me… but I felt like I was not doing the thing that I needed to be doing, I was missing it.

Then, surgery day came. Well, let's talk a little about the night before. The night before surgery, I was traumatized. Sleep does not happen. I found myself crying most of the night. Fear of the unknown. They were taking a part of me, the part of me that had nourished my children, the part that I, as well as most women feel is one of the largest feminine attributes that men find attractive. So, the next question that terrified me was, what was this going to do to my marriage?!

They tell us that breast cancer can be extremely hard on marriages. I feared, just as every person out there probably does/did, will he still love me without my breast? The plan is for immediate reconstruction, but they also inform you of the failure rate. All of it can be overwhelming. And this is what I learned. It is okay to have those days. As long as you remember that in the end, if you stay positive, and remain in LOVE, the love you have with your family, the love you have with friends and most important, the love and peace you have in and with God, Love will win. The focus you find is not about the loss of your breast. It is about something so much deeper. It took two years for me to figure out that I lost something, but it was not anything that I could not live without.

I woke up the day of surgery knowing we had to be out of the house at 4:00 am. I needed to do a breathing treatment and take a shower. Similar in a weird way to when I had packed my bag when I was pregnant for the hospital trip, I packed a bag that was ready to go.

Can we quickly talk about the hibiclens. Hibiclens is this lovely cleanser they have you wash with before surgery. I do not know why they do not just have us wash with bleach.... Again, I digress, I finished showering, checked my bag to make sure that I had all that I would need for my stay, looked around the room wistfully, thinking to myself "how did I get on this ride and when can I get off?" I walked across the hall, went into Gehrig's room first, kissed his forehead, whispered I love you, he said "love you mom." Walked into Jackson's room and repeated the process. I then walked down the stairs. Numb.

 Off to the hospital we go (pre covid). I sent the boys to school. If I could do that again, I would have given THEM the choice. What do you want to do? Be home? Go to hospital? Hang out at their beloved aunt's house? They should have had the choice. My suggestion to you, let your loved ones in. It is not just the warrior who is going through the cancer. It is the whole family. If I had just opened up a little, some of the doubts and fears all of us had could have been shared. Then we all could have shared each other's burden, maybe making it lighter for each other.

Joining Pete and I at the hospital was Pete, my dad, Patrick, and finally, Emily.

The team came into my room in shifts. First the oncologist Dr. K, then the general surgeon, Dr. B, then the plastic surgeon Dr. R, neither of us had any idea how important Dr R would become, he became one of my strongest fighters, available anytime, for anything. Again, I may sound like a broken record, but you should feel like all the doctors on your team are in the dugout fighting with you, not looking to get traded.

There was a bit of prepping that happened, drawings on your body that you never thought you would see. I tried along with my daughter to joke our way through it. Then the nervous giggling starts, and then, you are stuck in a loop, awkward. It was our coping mechanism. Not everyone in the room joined in with our way of coping, they did not see the humor, but what is the saying, if you do not laugh, you will cry.

Next, off to surgery. I kissed my loved one's goodbye, I remember really looking at their faces, wanting to remember everything about them. My dad trying to keep it together, and failing, my husband and son strong and silent, and my Emily, doing her best to be lighthearted. And off I went… but I knew I was not alone. I remember being rolled down the hall, and I cannot explain it, but I felt a presence. They moved me from the gurney to the operating room gurney. Again, I was scrubbed down, because the bleach, I mean hibiclens I did was not enough. I remember looking up at the bright light above me, they told me to count backwards. I said Hail Mary. I did not get far before I was asleep.

The next thing I remember is the recovery room, surgery had lasted about five hours. Feeling very groggy, I remember asking how and where my family was. I was genuinely concerned with how my dad was, really, I was concerned with how everyone was. I was told I could see them in a little bit. I do not know how much later, but I saw my beautiful husband's face over me as well as my dad's. My poor dad. He lost my mom in 1998. I knew being in the hospital was giving him terrible flashbacks. Only the person who was always by his side, me, was now on the table. I later found out from my daughter, that when the nurse came in and said, "only two of you can go back at a time," my dad stood up and looked like he would fight somebody for one of the spots. All I know is the two men who have had my heart for the longest were in front of me. I had woken up, and that was what mattered now.

I finally got to see my Patrick and my Emily. I cannot tell you what it feels like to see your loved one's faces after surgery. But it is close to heaven on earth. Again, if I could have a do over, I would have asked Pete to bring Gehrig and Jackson up. I needed them, and they needed me as well. I thought I was protecting them, but the most important thing they needed was to see that their mom had made it through surgery.

I started sending my family home. I hoped to be sleeping, and they had been at the hospital with me since before the sun came up, then you add the stress of the surgery hours, the waiting, my loved ones needed rest. Sure enough, I was sleepy that day, but that night the pain kicked in. If you have had a mastectomy with reconstruction, you will know what I am talking about. I remember no matter which way I moved, no matter what I did, I could not find a comfortable position. Just when I would doze off, a nurse would come in to take my vitals, so getting rest was not going to happen.

Emily and Pete showed up in the morning and I was very alert considering the lack of sleep. The nurse had already gone over some things with us. But not all. This may sound crazy, but we had questions. I do not know how we missed asking this question, but we wanted to know if I had anything left. They are sometimes able to save the nipples and we wanted to know if they had been able to do that. I was wrapped up like a Halloween mummy, so we could not look and see a thing. I also had this "chicken cutlet" like contraption on, that sucked the air out. It was a wound vacuum. It sounded like I was passing gas every few minutes. As soon as Emily and I realized what it sounded like, and a silence in the room occurred, it sent us into giggles. I had to wear this thing for the week, I was going to charm everyone I was around me. What could anyone say to me if they thought I was passing gas? Nobody would say a word, but my embarrassment was going to be through the roof. Well Dr. R. The plastic surgeon finally came in and she and I beat around the bush, not sure how to ask the question of the nipples. So, Emily just bursts out and asks, "does she have nipples or is she a barbie now?" Dr R. never having been a girl had no idea what that meant, any self-respecting Barbie girl knows that Barbie does not have nipples. We had to explain, and he smiled, but then went back to serious and said, "we had to take everything."

Again, I tried to find the silver lining. I was sitting up. My girl was hanging out with me. And we had nurse Karen of whom I was very fond, she had a hook up for Jell-O, and who does not like Jell-O? The following day, nurse Karen came in and said, "Claudia, if you get up and walk around, we will let you go home." I said, "how many times? I am in." Well, I had only been walking to and from the bathroom, so I looked at Pete and Emily and said, "let's get moving," so up I got. We managed to get my robe on, which with an IV and all my new hook ups was no small feat. And off to the races we went. We walked down our hall, turned left. As we were approaching the elevators, I saw to my horror I was on the oncology floor and threw a fit. Now everyone, think about this for a minute. I just had my cookies removed, undeniable pain I am in, and what am I upset about? That they put me, a breast cancer patient, on the oncology floor! Well, as I am bickering with my beloved and ever understanding husband and daughter about the floor I am on, Emily finally looks at me and says, "mom, you are a cancer patient." That shut me up pretty quick. I put my head as high as my surgical situation would allow, and kept on my walk, making sure to stop at both sides of the nurses' station so they saw that I went all the way around.

I then went back to my room and waited. I was ready to go. Boy, I had NO IDEA what I was in for when I got home.

Chapter Two: Let The Walk Begin

One of the first things the doctors tell you after you are diagnosed is not to google. Well, what did all of us do…google. Gratefully, my search led me to a reputable site, The American Cancer Society website. I found out about all the important work they do, and realized this is it.

What was it I was supposed to be doing? I felt a draw but could not put a finger on it. Then it hit me, so hard. It was staring at me, in front of me on the computer screen. I started researching how to do it. But I doubted it. Could I? Should I? What am I referring to? I started the Walking Warriors Chicago Strides Team. And I became possessed.

I called my daughter and said, "do you think you could help me?" She, like me, likes to plan things. I then recruited my husband. Without the two of them, I never would have gotten the team off the ground. I do not know if they truly realize how much I depended on their support, but it was everything to me. Patrick, Gehrig, and Jackson all did what they were able to do to help.

With Strides for Life, I found a purpose, a way to help, to maybe take a bite out of the thing that was taking a bite out of me. I found a way to fight back.

I was going to raise money for the ACS and help people, people like me, who may one day not have to go through what I was looking at if we find a cure. And it began. We started the team. Picked the team's name and signed up, we then started raising money.

Organizing and planning, I was trying to figure out what I could do to raise funds. It was already August. The walk was in October. So much to do, so little time.

The first thing I did was reach out to my girlfriends who are fellow warriors. Unfortunately, I have a few. Kathy and Lucia were the first, and both immediately responded that they would take part with me. It is with deepest regret that I say that Lucia's beautiful mother Maria, taken far too soon, was a warrior like us who battled breast cancer.

Next, I reached out to dear friends and family. I cannot say enough about the love and support that came from so many people. I was, and I still am, surrounded by so much love. I also want to acknowledge that some of you may not have the same support that I have. It was another reason I became so determined to raise money for the ACS. The outreach that they provide such as volunteer drivers who take patients to appointments, hope house, a safe place to stay for patients when treatment is far from their homes. They provide what so many people who are going through cancer need, support and answers.

I figured I would have time to work on the fundraiser while I was laid up recovering from surgery. I had no idea of the road I had just jumped on. And something every cancer patient needs to know is that each journey is unique. We all have relatable stories, though. I am always taken back when I am having a conversation with a fellow warrior and we find that similar thread, many of us go through similar things but again, each story is different. We will talk more about the walk and the planning and amazing execution of it a little later.

Chapter Three: After Surgery

I am getting out! Emily and Pete and I headed home. Thank God Emily did her research. I am going to add a few more things as well. Amanda sent me a goodie bag. It contained a cushion that goes over your seatbelt and provides MUCH needed cushion over your surgical area. I still use it to this day.

Each bump that we went over, felt like I was going to lose something, or hurl, it was a rough ride, I did not look forward to car rides, and unfortunately, so many doctor appointments needed to be scheduled. We finally got home, I saw Gehrig and Jackson finally! And my sweet little yorkies, no need to pretend anymore, we all know Hampton was my buddy, and he truly became my tiny knight in shining armor. Thankfully, Emily had bought a wedge for the bed. Little did I know that getting in and out of bed was going to be a struggle. The wedge is an absolute necessity if you are going to be insistent as I was after that first surgery to sleep in my own bed. I also have a bedroom on the second floor. That became an issue as well, you see going up and down steps if you are the only one home is not ideal. The medicine. Oh, my goodness all the medicine, I felt like I was opening a pharmacy! And my family, amazing. They woke me up and made sure I did not miss a dose of anything.

I am going to share a favorite story of mine from this time. Our youngest, Jackson, was holding a lot of his emotions about my diagnosis to himself (I think all my children did). He played football for the local high school. I was determined to go to his game on Saturday…three days after I came home. I wanted him to see me in the stands, his biggest cheerleader. He did not know I was coming. They dropped me off, so I did not have to walk as far, thankfully we had no wait to get in, as we came after the game started. I wore a long maxi dress (so I could conceal the lines coming out of me, I had four balls that were draining, filled with blood, let's not forget the wound vacuum machine that made the farting sounds and my being wrapped like a mummy to conceal the hot mess that was my chest). I honestly thought going would be no big deal. Well, it was a bit more than I had expected, but watching Jackson on the field he loved so much made it all worth it. And I knew he saw me. He also took to wearing a pink armband for me. I also want to acknowledge all the football moms who supported not just me but took care of Jackson. Especially Polly, Daria, and our dear Jen who has since passed away. Two of these moms are breast cancer survivors who gave me helpful advice and guidance. Polly has joined me in recent years, I am so proud to have her walk with me on the Walking Warriors.

Jackson also played baseball, and I was friends with those moms. However, I had kept my diagnosis under wraps. I think like many cancer patients, we do not want people to pity us, look at us funny, or treat us differently. They must have caught wind through the grapevine. After the game let out, we were waiting for Jackson to come up from the tunnel. He came up quickly, a grin on his face, so happy to see me. Here is the thing I will never forget. Those baseball moms, whom I also love, came up and moved in on me with offers of help and support. Jackson did not even realize he did it, but he moved in front of me to protect me so these women he knew and trusted would not touch me in my delicate condition. He was protecting his Mama. My baby boy, as well as my other children, Patrick, Emily, and Gehrig had become my protectors. I do not know if he saw the tears in my eyes. I hope he did not think they were tears of pain. At that moment, the joy I had for my son, my youngest child protecting me like that, was another thing that made me look at the blessing around me.

Later that day, Pete decided to have a cookout. Patrick came in from Chicago. My dad, grandma and grandpa, my brother and sister-in-law (I say in-laws, but we really are one big extended family), Danny (who is like another brother to me) and his dad, who we all call Papa, were also present. As I say, I had played my cards close to the vest and asked the family to not put the word out about my cancer. At some point I looked at Papa, and he was trying to hide tears. He got up and came over, hugged me, and said, "I didn't know." This broke my heart, because this man who we have since lost, had lost his beloved wife to cancer. Cancer affects us all. Your cancer may affect others in ways you do not know, cancer has a way that makes people stop in their tracks. If you ask someone, they know someone else who has had cancer or has cancer. Its ugly fingers leave a mark. I know we were probably nuts having family over not just Saturday, but also Sunday. But I knew that these people I loved needed to see me as much as I needed to see them. Seeing my cousin and my auntie Judy (my mom's sister) was hard for me, maybe it's because whenever I am with my aunt, the void that has been left by my mom is so raw... I adore them, they are a constant reminder to me that mom is only as far as me closing my eyes.

Maybe some of you can relate to this, but when I found out I had cancer, I really tried to keep myself together. I allowed myself to cry in the shower, in my car, and the day after I found out... I drove to my mother's grave and laid on it. I drenched her headstone in tears. When I say, "I felt I wasn't alone," I know Jesus walked this journey and is still walking with me. But I believe my mom has been working overtime whispering in people's ears. My next bit of advice is to allow ALL the love in. If people offer it to you, take it. If people offer prayer, thank them, and ask how you can pray for them. It was through little daily graces I found my way:

The Barbie from1960's that my older cousin Patti sent me that we played with (really, I forced her to play with me) along with a note, saying I needed to give this to my granddaughter someday.

The bible I could draw in from my other cousin, Geralyn, which allowed me to read verses and do artwork, two things I love doing.

The cards that came from my Religious Ed class telling me they were praying for me and wishing me well.

My best friends, who are sisters to me. There, always.

My daughter number 2 calling to check in.

Daughter number 2(you share this Katie and Jess) making me my warrior welcome sign.

My daughter working from home (and her amazing boss, Erik. allowing that so she could take care of me).

Erik designing the Walking Warriors shirt (and sneaking my initials in, I just found that out recently) … the best.

My niece and sis baking for me and I know praying so hard.

My cousin, Audrey, and my Aunt Judy, came to visit with thoughtful gifts, one so very perfect, a disk full of photos of family and friends, especially my mom as a child.

The flowers and texts.

Patrick calling when I knew how busy he was.

Gehrig and Jackson being available for me, offering to get things, help with things… giving hugs that teenagers are so fond of doing (laughing).

My dad and Kerry driving miss Claudia.

And Pete trying to hold it all together and making his Jackson coined "struggle meals."

Every single person reached who reached out, to me, to Pete or one of the family. All the people who looked after my family. Thank you!

The amazing care team that I had. How can I thank all of you! From Dr M. my radiologist, Dr K and his entire staff, special shout out to NP Amie, she was and is one of my favorite humans. Dr R, nurse Jamie and his whole staff, I will never be able to thank you for all that you did and do.

What I know is without the prayers, and so much more from so many I just don't know where and what I would have done.   I can never thank you enough.

Chapter Four: Your Family

My husband had a lot going on in his head. Men tend to hold it ALL in and I hope that someday they can learn that expressing emotion is not a sign of weakness. WE learned together that he was having all the same fears I was, However, we did not learn this until 2021, three years after I was diagnosed. But as all men are taught to do, he was strong for me. He was strong for all of us. I now look back and think his own mental health suffered because of holding it all in.

Another suggestion, seek help with any signs of distress in any family member. I wish that it would be mandatory for all families to go through therapy. No one can be prepared for what happens when a family member is diagnosed. The head and mind go right to places that remind me of the older woman in St Elmo's Fire at the dinner table who has to whisper "cancer."

I honestly feel couples should openly discuss their fears together, because most of the trouble really stems from fear. Fear of change, fear of the unknown, fear of the future! Couples, as well as family members, would be able to offer more support to one another.

And then there are the children. The kids in my case managed it each in their own way. I feel the worst for Emily. I was afraid to let Pete see my chest until it healed. I again say therapy may have helped us navigate this. So poor Emily was put in the position to be my caretaker. And because we were all powering through, I had no idea Pete, instead of feeling a sense of relief, was feeling a bit left out. But again, after I saw my chest, that looked like someone had taken a baseball bat to it, I could not let him see me like that. Then as if things could not get worse... I went necrotic, what this means is my skin started to die, it was not anything anyone could imagine. So, I landed back in surgery in short order to try and debride the area, hopefully remove the dead area so that the healthy skin would start to heal. I go home and start recovery again, but I am feeling terrible that everyone is taking time off. So, I send everyone to work knowing full well I am running a fever. But I thought I could handle it. I was also using a medication to try and stop the necrosis that made me terribly nauseous. By the time everyone came home, I was in tears, could not move and was running a fever so high I am embarrassed to say the degrees. Needless to say, an immediate call was placed to the doctor, and I know both Pete and Emily wanted to throttle me, but I think they felt so bad for me they didn't have the heart.

Back to the hospital we go. Another surgery. In the end. It all had to come out. My body was just so angry, and I was worn out. Cultures were taken and I had an infection, followed by a seroma, at this point I was going in about every two weeks for surgery. And guess what? One of the surgeries was a couple of days before the walk, and come hell or high water, I was walking.

At this point, our team Walking Warriors had grown to at least forty people and that is how many people we had walking on our beloved Lake Front. My cousin and her husband came from Ohio, and I think she felt good coming to see us. It's so hard being far away from family when anything good or bad happens. She came with chicken soup and all the fixings.

The day of the walk, we put on our special t-shirts that Emily's boss man, Erik designed. The sun had not even come up. But this day I felt like I was going to conquer the world. It was my mom's birthday. We put my tutu on, that Emily and I had found to hide the drains and all the other good things (we all know these things are not good, but necessary). Emily made food, we had everyone over for breakfast so we could head out together.

The doorbell rang, and my sister-in-law Kerry, is standing there with a pink wagon with my other sister-in-law, Julie, who flew in from New Hampshire to surprise me…. with my niece Caroline and my nephew Eric, I again find myself in tears, I would like to mention that Caroline's boyfriend, was there as well (what is amazing, this young couple will soon be married, and I get to watch it, another milestone I can chalk up!). I know how much this means to Julie. She has lost loved ones to this disease already, and this hits so close to home for her. The joy I have as I stand there knowing I have sprung a leak from one of my drains, nothing matters. I'm wearing a pink tutu, and nothing else matters. We were going to make a stand against cancer. We were all going to be together and that is what happened.

We arrived at Soldier Field, gathered, and two pink heads came walking toward me. Patrick and Amanda. I am overjoyed. This girl got my engineer of a son to wear a pink wig! Imagine looking out, seeing the amazing lake shore that Chicago has to offer, and everywhere you turn is a sea of pink. Every person surrounding you is there for the sole purpose of supporting Strides for Life. There to either honor a loved one walking or a loved one lost. You might think being there is sad, but it is not. For me, it was a moment of triumph. I walked, I sat in the pink wagon, I was surrounded by that love I keep talking about. So many photos that day. A day of triumph for all of us warriors and our families.

Since that first year. We have raised over $50,000 for ACS. Every year, we add the names of loved ones diagnosed and loved ones lost to all types of cancer. My dad joined us Warriors last year with a colon cancer diagnosis. This year more names will be added, and more than one beloved is gone from this disease. Last year we honored Maria, Lucia's mom, and a woman named Sharon. This lady will never know how much she inspired me, she inspired me so much… I went back to school to get my degree in psychology. Last year's shirt was her art, and I was so proud to walk wearing it.

Some years ago, we were still in our early forties when a classmate of ours lost her battle to breast cancer. Her son was still in elementary school at the time. When my daughter was in kindergarten, her best friend Noelle lost her mom to breast cancer. It affected me, at the time I especially remember having this need to want to do something for their children. What I know is this, as bad as I felt for these families, it really doesn't hit you, until it hits your house.

When it comes to your family, my best advice is to pay attention. Don't be afraid to ask for professional help or to seek the help of your pastor.

What difference does it make if you survive the cancer, and your family falls apart? It is never too late to seek help. You making yourself better will always make your circumstances better. Now let's talk about that.   Not all relationships survive the stress of cancer. Relationships are hard, and nothing can put a relationship to the test like this disease. But you are never alone. God may close a door, but the window will open. Reach out, ask for help. Ask, don't let pride be the thing that takes you out. There are resources. Again, counseling is often available, ask your doctor, and reach out to your church. The American Cancer Society is another resource to use. You have people, you must have faith it will be as it should, all in His time. Not ours.

Remember also sometimes, we pick our family. I am fortunate enough to have friends who are family. Remember, many times people don't want to bother you, and sometimes you have to ask for help. And it is OKAY.

My final surgery was on our wedding anniversary 7/26/2019. I feel blessed because as had become the norm for all the other surgeries, I was not alone when I closed my eyes. The loving presence of Jesus always surrounded and protected me. We all waited anxiously to see if all would "take." It did and that part of my journey is over.

I am almost five years post diagnosis. I am waiting to hear the words from my oncologist, "you are released." But one thing is certain. No matter what, cancer did not win. I won.

In the end, the fundraiser was truly a success, and still is because of an army of family and friends who are family. If you ever feel like you have no control, think about raising money for the cause. I can't explain the gratification of helping others. I know when I'm gone, I will have made a mark, I hope I have shown my children that there is more than one way to fight, and that no one fights alone. I hope I showed them that I was not and will not be defined by cancer. Even if you do nothing more than fight this fight, you will have made a mark on everyone around you. Remember you are enough.

Chapter Five: The Future

So here I am today, five years a survivor and thriver. I have not fully been released. But that is okay.

Here is what has happened: Gehrig graduated high school and went off to Purdue just like his big brother, Patrick; his sister, Emily; and his cousins, Ben, Eric, and Caroline. My other nephews Brett and Mathew have graduated college and moved to various places in their lives, and I have watched it all.

Jackson graduated high school and he is at Purdue as well. He, like all the kids, is a testament to hard work and determination. Both Gehrig and Jackson dealt with covid during some defining moments. They learned to pivot. They had to learn that early. But I am proud of them for doing it. I can't wait to see what these two young ones of mine accomplish.

Emily, my beloved girl. Is thriving at her job. She is the epitome of loyalty and beauty. Many moons ago my mom told me amid her and I having a heated disagreement she said, "Claudia, someday I will be the best friend you could ever have" I didn't understand that until after I had Patrick, that understanding of "unconditional love' that a parent has for a child. She was my best friend, and I am honored that my child/children are now some of my "best friends'.

Patrick, he married his girl, Amanda. And let me tell you of the happy tears that rolled down that day. I look at the pictures and photographer managed to catch me weeping a lot. What many did not realize is I had managed to tick off a significant amount from the list I had given to the oncologist. The graduation parties happened, I danced with Pete (and Patrick, who himself is a miracle) at Patrick and Amandas wedding. We now have another daughter I did not have to work or pay for (grinning). I am living my life to the best of my ability.

Will the fear of reoccurrence ever go away for any of us? I don't think so. I think it lives in the back of our mind. But to the best of my ability in this covid world, we try and live our lives.

It took many surgeries, and I will not say how many, because your journey is not mine.

What I can tell you is, I finally figured out to get a recliner so that getting up was not traumatizing.

What I learned is alternative therapy to compliment traditional is immensely helpful and should be considered if offered and taken and I thank Amie and Pam for all they did for me as well as those at the Cancer Resource Center.

If your gut is telling you to get a second opinion, do it.

If you need to, hold someone's hand. Chances are that person needs to hold your hand just as much. You could be giving comfort just as you are receiving it.

Be patient with treatment/ therapy. If you trust your doctor, trust the process.

Join a support group. There are so many available. Church, Hospitals, ACS,

Keep a journal. It helps keep your mind straight, and it's a good place to jot questions you may have for one doctor or another.

Yoga does the body good. You can adjust it for all cancers to fit where you are. Locally we have "The Cancer Resource Center" an amazing resource for cancer patients.

Walk.

If you get lymphedema, seek help, get sleeves and gloves and ask for a referral from a therapist who works specifically on lymphedema patients.

If you have any questions, ask for help from your providers, that is why they are there.

Cancer is not the end. We are called Warriors for a reason.

I wish you love and blessings, from our house to yours.

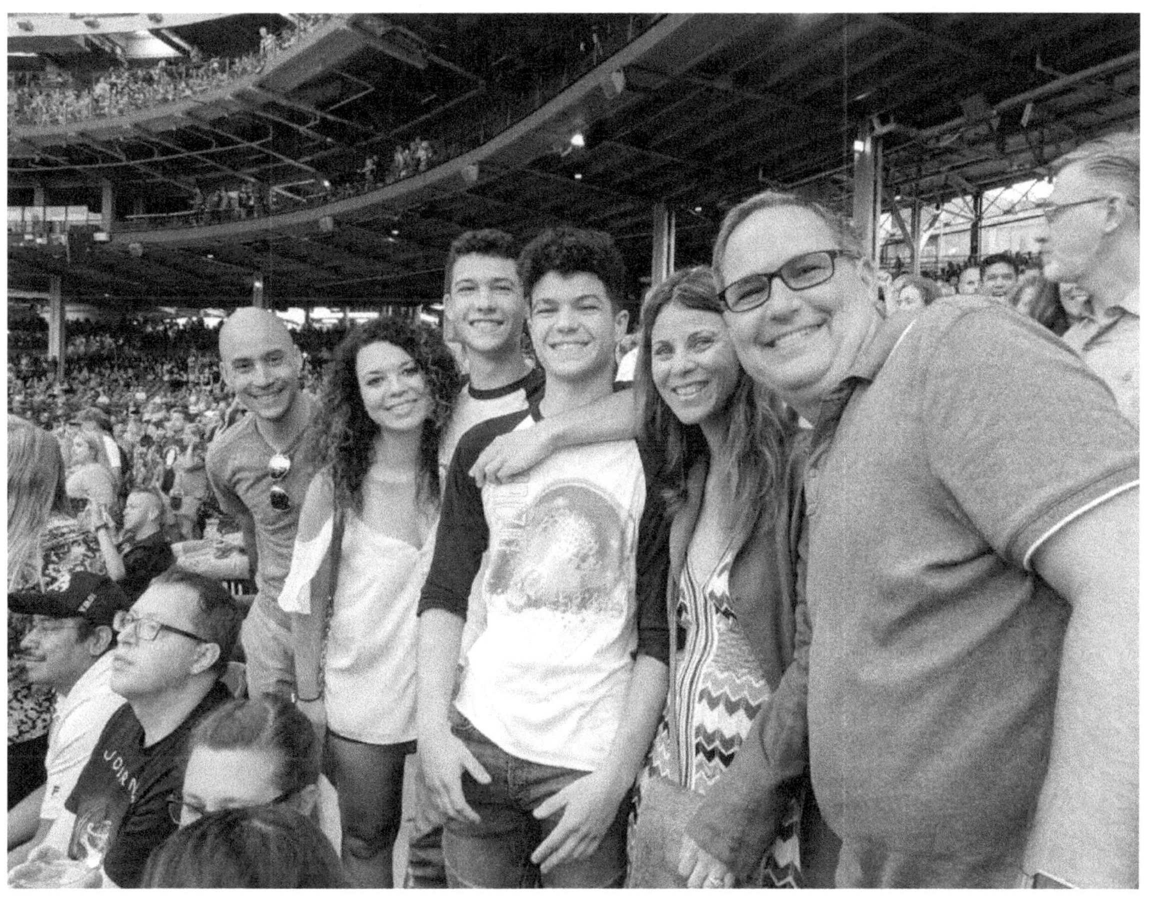

July of 2018 The Def Leppard/Journey concerts

Patrick, Emily, Gehrig, Jackson, Me, Pete

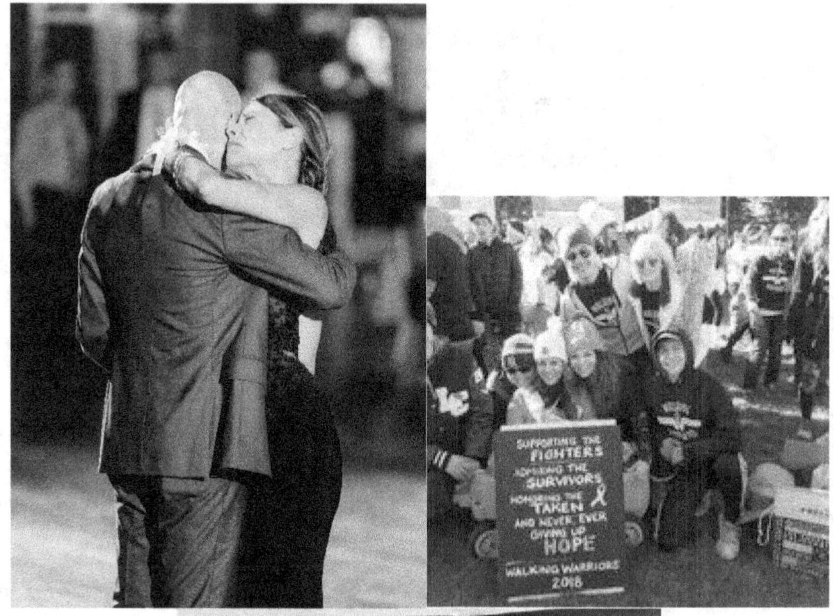

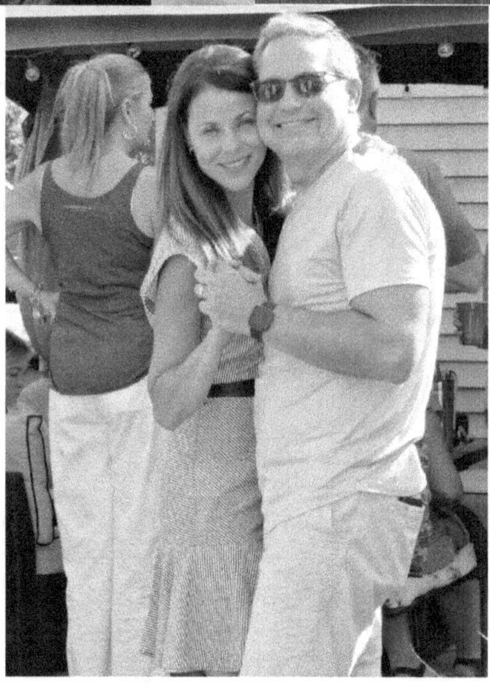

Epilogue/Conclusion

I hope you find something useful in my cancer journey. I have felt for a long time I needed to share, as so often when we are going through this we are utterly alone. I wish someone had told me just a few of the things I think BC patients should know. In the end you are not alone.

Bibliography

Acknowledgments

I would like to thank my husband, my partner of 31 years. You stood by me when I was at my lowest. It is because of you I smile each morning, the air I breathe. By the grace of God, we were brought to each other so long ago. I pray for many healthy, blessed years with you... enjoying all that life has to offer us. Can't wait to be Duchess and Comish

To our children, God entrusted us with you. Every day, Dad and I pray we do right by and for you. Know You are loved more than all the stars in the sky. You make our world spin. Amanda, thank you for making our child so incredibly happy, we are blessed by you.

My beloved mom (gone too soon) and Dad, you have always been by my side. The good, the bad. Your strength taught me how to fight this, you taught me how to love unconditionally. My first loves

To my sisters, you know who you are. You encourage and support. Your worlds could be upside down, yet you still give, I hope that I provide that same support for you.

G and G. Thank you for always being there for us. Grandpa, you showed us how to fight this past year. We are so glad you are here with us.

To my Gram little do you know. My whole life. It is you who showed me the most powerful love of Jesus. You were an amazing example and the love that you spilled on all of us, I still feel today. Mom and auntie Judy are so like you it is crazy.

To my brothers Rick, Benjamin and Michael. The good, the bad. I love you. Ben, you are missed every day. I hope all of you are proud of me.

About the Author

Claudia J Sarbieski was born in Chicago on the 16 May 1968,

Claudia is happily married to her husband Peter of 31 years and the mother to their four children Patrick (Amanda), Emily, Gehrig and Jackson

Claudia recently and joyously went back to school to earn her degree in psychology with the hope of someday helping cancer patients and their families.

Mrs. Sarbieski was diagnosed with breast cancer in 2018 and started fundraising for the ACS the same year under Walking Warriors.